THE LICE-BUSTER BOOK

What To Do When Your Child
Comes Home With Head Lice!

by Lennie Copeland

Illustrations by
Ashley Copeland Griggs

PUBLISHED BY
AUTHENTIC PICTURES
MILL VALLEY, CALIFORNIA

Copyright © 1995 by Lennie Copeland
First Printing 1995
Printed in the United States of America

10 9 8 7 6 5 4 3 2 1

Library of Congress Cataloging-in-Publication Data
Copeland, Lennie.
    The Lice-Buster Book: What to Do When Your Child
    Comes Home With Head Lice / by Lennie Copeland;
    with illustrations by Ashley Copeland Griggs.

    1. Lice
    2. Pediculosis
    3. Health – Child
    ISBN 1-885883-11-0
    Library of Congress Catalogue Number 94-96323

This book does not guarantee that all readers will be able to completely eliminate lice from their lives by following the steps advised herein. It is meant simply to serve as the best assembly of information known to date about the habits of lice and the most effective procedures for killing lice and nits.

Published by **Authentic Pictures**
                89 Walnut Avenue
                Mill Valley, CA 94941

Cover design and production by Jill Davey, JPD Communications, Berkeley, CA
Interior design and production by Lory Poulson Graphic Arts, Richmond, CA

for Ashley and Ian

ACKNOWLEDGMENTS

A book like this requires few acknowledgements because there are few who know anything about lice. So I am in great debt to Professors David Taplin and Terri Meinking at the University of Miami School of Medicine, for their hard work researching lice and willingness to share their expertise, answer my questions, and review a draft of the book.

I also thank John Poorbaugh, ectoparasite specialist retired from the California Department of Health Services and Dr. Dennis Juranek, an expert on pediculosis at the Centers for Disease Control, Andy Sopchak at Burroughs Wellcome, and pharmacist Steve Bacon of Lawson-Dyer Pharmacy, for many hours discussing lice and the various treatments.

Two nurses who deal with lice in the schools reviewed a draft of the book and I thank them for their help: Trish Bascom, Head Nurse in the San Francisco Unified School District and Ann Solomon, Head Nurse of the Mill Valley School District, in California. I also thank Bridget Ward, PhN, Los Angeles County Department of Health Services for the information she provided.

Several schools participated in a survey of the lice problem among their students. They wish to remain anonymous, but are thanked for their vital help. Shirley Freeman, Director of Kittredge School, is particularly thanked for her open, immediate and enthusiastic assistance with the survey in her school.

Most of all, I thank my children, Ashley (12) and Ian (7) for lending me their heads and cooperating so patiently with my research. May they remain lice-free forevermore!

TABLE OF CONTENTS

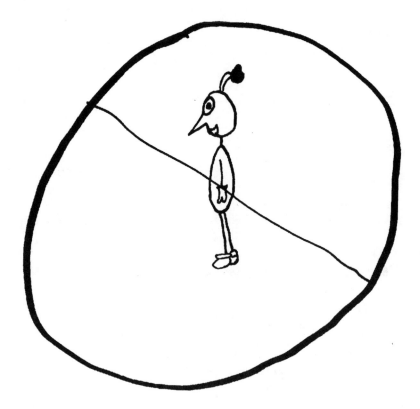

INTRODUCTION

Why a book about head lice? Because every year 10–12 million children get lice. If you bought this book because you are dealing with head lice in your own family or school, rest assured, you are not alone. Pediculosis (presence of lice) strikes more children than all other communicable childhood diseases combined, excluding the common cold. The schools are in a state of perpetual lice alert. Health professionals say the problem is endemic and epidemic. Pharmaceutical firms report double digit increases in sales of pediculicides, up to 19% growth. Meanwhile, many of you who must deal with lice are at your wits end.

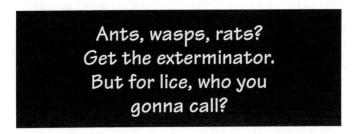

Ants, wasps, rats?
Get the exterminator.
But for lice, who you
gonna call?

Unfortunately, frantic parents and school personnel have had nowhere to turn for reliable information about what to do about head lice. There are no books on the subject and only scant information in public health agency brochures that always advise, "Consult your pediatrician." But most pediatricians don't know any more about lice than the average parent, and many know less. After all, doctors don't study lice in medical school.

Of course, there are the occasional back-to-school articles about lice, offering the same outdated, unhelpful, and even incorrect information that is recycled in health department brochures, school hand-outs, and pharmaceutical packaging. To make matters worse, the instructions on lice treatments are often unclear and incomplete, resulting in misuse, reinfestation, and secondary complications. It seems nobody really knows much about lice. Myths abound, parents rely on folklore, and lice flourish.

How can it be that so little is known about such a widespread problem? One reason is that lice are not a reportable disease so health agencies have no mechanism for epidemiological study. Moreover, lice are not a popular subject for scientific research because head lice cannot be cultivated off the human head and few researchers are willing to raise lice on their own bodies. Rumor has it that most lice researchers are divorced!

Thankfully, there is a handful of committed researchers around the world who are willing to put lice on themselves for what they matter-of-factly call "blood meals." One group is the Field Epidemiology Survey Team at the University of Miami School of Medicine. Professors David Taplin and Terri Meinking have been studying lice all over the world. Many of their findings on the habits of head lice have been included in this book.

THE LICE-BUSTER BOOK book aims to demythologize lice and to furnish the information you need to gain control of the lice problem in your community and your home. It provides step-by-step procedures for treating lice infestation. It also makes suggestions for schools because parents can't do it alone. A child can't be completely protected from lice except by isolation; as long as any children in an environment have lice, all are vulnerable.

Chances are the problem can't be completely eliminated: lice have survived since Neanderthal man. No treatment is guaranteed 100% effective and no amount of precaution can completely prevent head lice. One lousy louse may slip through. So this book can't guarantee you will never see another louse. But I do promise that if you follow the book precisely, you will see the end of the nerve-wracking, costly, time-consuming struggle with chronic lice infestations that threaten to drive you *mad!*

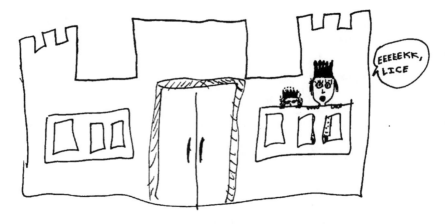

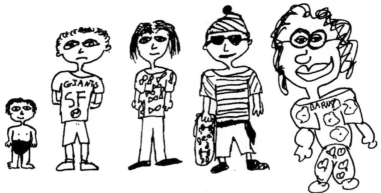

Anyone can get lice!

CHAPTER 1

Lice Styles of the Rich and Famous

THE STIGMA OF LICE

You've heard that head lice are no cause for shame and no reflection of the hygiene in your home. But when you find lice in your family, you are horrified. You're first thought (or shriek) is "Oh my God!" Suddenly your own head starts to itch. In fact, it may itch at the mere mention of lice. You may itch all the way through this book!

Deep down inside, you are repulsed by lice. You also feel lice are unclean and only unclean children get lice. Actually, this is not true. As one expert states, "Dirt does not cause lice to appear on a child's scalp." Lice are no more inclined to reside in unclean conditions than they are to live on the heads of well-scrubbed children. In fact, if they show any prejudice at all, lice do not like dirt and prosper more readily on a clean scalp rather than a neglected one.

> Dirt does not cause lice to appear on a child's scalp.

ANYONE CAN GET LICE

Anyone can get lice. Children in the best schools and upper crust families get lice. Children of celebrities get lice. In one of the most exclusive schools in San Francisco, California, 17 out of 22 girls in one class were found to have lice. When a child comes home with lice, it is virtually inevitable

Lice favor children between 5 and 12 in all races except black. their siblings will be infested too, even infants and frequently their parents. Again, hygiene has nothing to do with it.

Certain groups do tend to get lice more than others. The highest concentration is among children between the ages of 5 and 12, in all races except African Americans, who almost never get lice. In study after study, prevalence of lice infestation was 30 to 36 times higher in whites than in American blacks in the same school classes.

Girls have a slightly greater tendency to get lice than boys. This has less to do with hair length than the hair mass since density of hair makes it harder to find and remove nits.

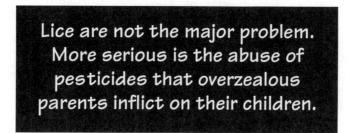

Lice are not the major problem. More serious is the abuse of pesticides that overzealous parents inflict on their children.

It's important to dismiss any notions of a stigma attached to lice because *the presence of lice is not the major problem.* A much more serious problem is the panic and abuse of pesticides that overzealous parents might inflict on their children in their frenzy to eliminate them. Lice treatments, euphemistically called "medication" or "shampoo," are pesticides and some of them are toxic. Parents who would never in a million years put ant or roach killer on their children's heads don't think twice about soaking their child's head in lice treatments. So the most important message of this book is this: *Do not go wild and overdo any treatment.* Lice can be effectively treated by following the instructions in this book.

IT'S A LOUSY SITUATION ALL AROUND

In the mid 1970's the U.S. Center for Disease Control found increasing rates of head lice infestation. Among the children surveyed in three cities, infestation ranged from 3% to 20%. In some areas, lice infest as many as 40% of non-black school children. Even without current data, public health officials agree there has been a sharp increase in the frequency of head lice in the United States in all socioeconomic classes.

No region is free from lice infestation, although prevalence rates vary. Lice are most concentrated in New York, California, Florida, Southern Texas and the border states.

Head lice infestations have increased in all classes in the United States.

Infestation is seasonal in New England but year-round in the South and West. Lice infestations peak in November for the West and in September for the Northeast, North Central and South. Lice also seem to be a greater problem in cosmopolitan areas than in rural or suburban, possibly because of crowding which enables the spread of lice.

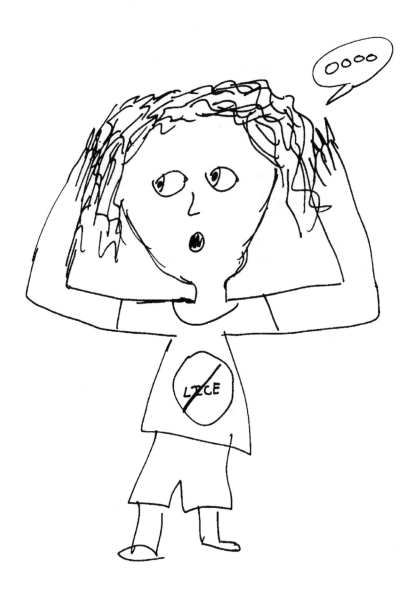

How I feel with lice . . . Ashley, age 12

WHY NIT PICK?

Many children, faced with yet another lice shampoo will protest, "So what if I have lice! I *like* lice!"

Good question. Lice are generally more unpleasant for the parent than the child. So, why not spare the child and just leave the lice alone? Here's why: lice can spread to enormous numbers of people and cause much bodily discomfort to those infested. The itching is a major irritation and the general stress of the condition can cause a child to be inattentive, restless, distractable, and listless at school. In short, they feel "lousy" as a result of their lice.

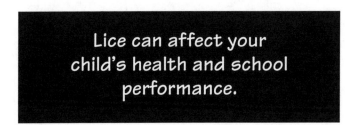

Lice can affect your child's health and school performance.

In severe cases, an infested child may become lethargic, literally a "nit-wit." The child may develop a mild fever, muscular aches, and swollen glands in the neck and/or under the arms. Children with lice show a significant increase in the frequency of conjunctivitis — although conjunctivitis may be the result not of infestation but repeated use of certain lice treatments. In cases of long duration, the hair may become matted by foul-smelling, oozing pus.

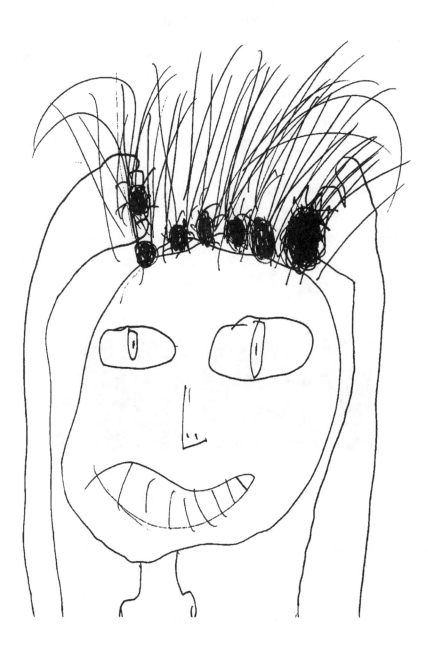

How I feel with lice . . . Ian, age 6

LICE AND DISEASE

Heavy infestations of lice may cause intense skin irritation; scratching may lead to scraping the skin and secondary infections. Constant scratching with unclean hands may cause bacterial infection leading to boils, impetigo, and inflammation of the lymph nodes at the neck.

Whether lice can actually spread disease has been somewhat controversial. Scientists do know that as lice travel from scalp to scalp, they can carry on their feet the streptococcal bacteria. The human body louse (a critter distinct from the head louse) spread typhus that caused colossal mortality of the troops during World War I and II. In recent cases of bubonic plague lice have been suspected as a likely carrier, but without solid evidence. Today head lice are not considered to be disease carriers, but Professor David Taplin at the University of Miami School of Medicine, Department of Dermatology, says it is unclear if head lice spread disease only because the question has not been researched.

Some people have voiced concern that lice might be able to spread AIDS, but this is highly doubtful. There was a similar scare about mosquitos, which proved to be nonsense. Besides, most lice travel within the 5–12 year old age group, which is not generally sexually active nor likely to have AIDS. The U.S. National Institutes for Health recently invited scientists to study the question.

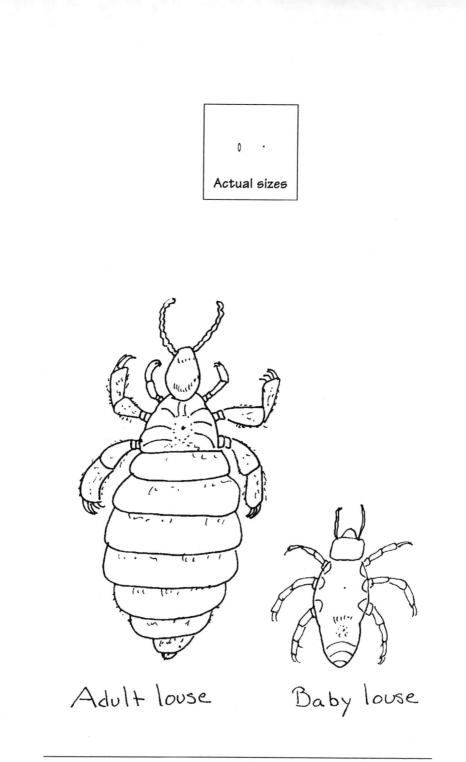

Actual sizes

Adult louse

Baby louse

CHAPTER 2
The Facts of Lice

OF LICE AND MEN

Lice (order Pthiraptera) are small, parasitic insects divisible into two main groups: Mallophaga, the biting lice, and Anoplura, the sucking lice. There are about 2,900 known species of Mallophaga and about 400 species of Anoplura.

Probably all species of birds have lice and most mammals. You may be greatly relieved by this bit of news: none have been found on the duckbilled platypus, anteaters, armadillos, bats or whales.

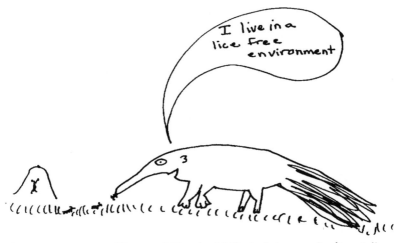

Anteaters, armadillos and the duckbilled platypus don't get lice.

Within suborder Anoplura are three species of lice that are regularly found on man: pediculus corporus (body lice), pediculus capitis (head lice), and Phthirus pubis (pubic lice or "crabs").

GENERAL FEATURES

Head lice are smaller than a sesame seed. They are wingless with flattened bodies ranging in size from 2.4 mm to 3 mm in females; the males are generally somewhat smaller than the females. They have six legs equipped with claws to grasp the hair and skin.

Lice take on the color of their background, greyish white on Europeans, blackish on Africans and other dark-skinned races. Depending on the hair coloring, they may be whitish, yellow, brown, or black. This is why they are so hard to find, particularly since they flee light and hide behind strands of hair.

MY, HOW THEY DO TRAVEL

Lice do not jump, hop or fly. But they do get around, moving from head to head (or from head to pillow to head) with an astonishing ease, particularly among younger children who tend to play closely together. They also spread more quickly in the winter because of shared hats and coats hung together.

A louse can travel 1 inch in five seconds.

Movements of lice are haphazard, though they are attracted by body heat and humidity. They meander in all directions but under optimal conditions a louse can travel 1 inch in five seconds and can cover long distances (e.g., 15 feet) in this meandering fashion. In certain circumstances, one single louse could easily visit several heads in one day.

LOUSY HABITS

Head lice live on the human scalp, and only on humans.
They do not live on pets. On girls they prefer the scalp at the
nape of the neck or behind the ears and on boys they tend
towards the top of the head. In both boys and girls, lice can
be found all over the head.

Lice live by biting and sucking blood from the human
scalp. The louse finds a nice spot on the head, grabs the skin
with its teeth, and thrusts three miniscule "straws" into the
scalp. One of these straws injects saliva full of anticoagulant
and one probes for a blood vessel. When found, it pierces the
blood vessel and sucks the blood while the anticoagulant keeps
the blood from clotting. Lice will feed for 45 seconds about
every two to three hours, each leaving between 8–12 *bites* in
the course of one day.

LIFE CYCLE OF A LOUSE

The process begins when two kids lean
over a book together, exchange hats, or share a
brush or comb. An adult female louse crawls
from one head to the other and proceeds to lay
up to 10 eggs a day for about a week.

A louse can lay 10 eggs each day.

The eggs of head lice are called *nits*. The tiny yellowish
white or grayish white nits are shaped like a tear drop, mea-
suring 0.8 mm. Freshly laid, they are transparent and blend in
with all colors of hair so they are hard to see. The female

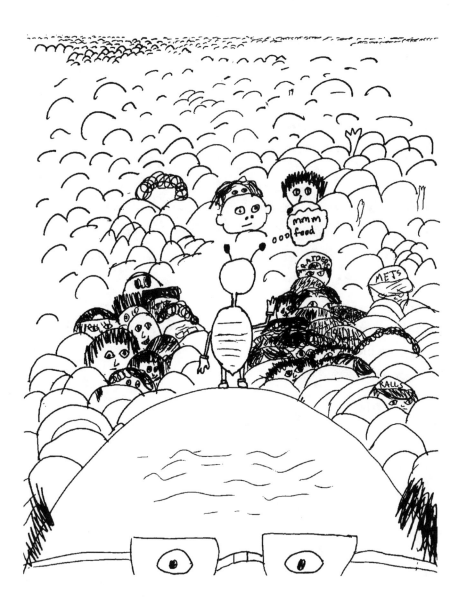

Lice have a blood meal every two to three hours

attaches the nits to the hair with a glue-like substance that makes it nearly impossible to remove the nits. Ordinary combing, brushing or shampooing will not shake them.

Eggs hatch in about one week to ten days, depending on the particular lice population and environmental conditions such as warmth of the scalp. For example, the eggs on a child's head in the summer in a warm climate will hatch sooner than eggs on a child's head in the winter in a cold climate, unless the homes are well heated and children bundled.

When the egg hatches, an immature louse, called a nymph, emerges. At birth the only pigment is in the eyes and claws. Otherwise the louse is uncolored, transparent and the size of the period at the end of this sentence. In short, virtually invisible.

The nymph immediately sets about hunting for blood. As the louse fills its gut with blood it turns bright red, so it becomes a tiny red dot. It will still be hard to find but at least now it is visible.

The young louse molts three times in the next 9 days, becoming slightly larger with each molt. It is mature after the third molt, normally within seven to ten days after hatching.

When reaching maturity, the louse begins its own family. Thus the entire life cycle, from egg to egg, is just about two weeks: one week in the egg sack and one week to reach maturity and begin laying eggs. (It's actually more like eight days each, but a week is easier to remember.) An adult will live for up to 30 days.

REPRODUCTION MATHEMATICS

One louse can lay 300 eggs in a month.

The average female louse produces between 200 to 300 eggs in her life-span, over 90% which will hatch successfully if not treated or removed.

If one adult louse lays ten eggs a day for 30 days, each egg which hatches and begins to lay eggs in just two weeks, and *those* eggs hatch and lay eggs in two weeks — you can see how a child could be infested with a swarm of lice after just a month or two.

Fortunately, some sort of population control limits lice infestations. Most people find only a few adult lice — up to a dozen — but many more nits. Counts over 100 are uncommon.

SURVIVAL OFF THE HOST

Head lice spend their entire life cycle, from egg to adult, on a host. The louse usually dies within a day off the human scalp, but may live as long as two days depending on conditions. Researchers have found no lice living beyond 48 hours without a human blood meal.

The louse is adapted to maintain close human contact. Being attracted by body heat and repelled by light, it stays within the warmth and darkness of the hosts hair. However, lice do leave their hosts to pass to another host of the same species: your kid's sibling, classmate, or you.

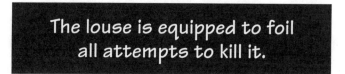

The louse is biologically engineered to protect itself against attempts to destroy it. The egg is attached with a glue that so far has been resistant to solvents. Lice quickly shut down their respiratory passages if immersed in water, so you can't drown them. They also attempt to shut down when a pediculicide is applied.

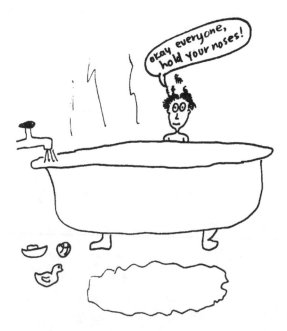

Lice shut down their systems for survival

I thought I discovered a treatment for lice when I dropped a blob of tree tea oil shampoo on a louse and it stopped moving after a few minutes. I rinsed it off and nothing happened: it looked deader than a doornail. I forgot about it, but ten minutes later I noticed my little louse was crawling along its strand of hair as if nothing had happened. It had simply "played dead" for ten minutes. The moral of the story is this: a listless louse is not necessarily dead!

THE TALE OF THE DEAD NIT

Just about anybody will tell you that lice lay only one egg to a shaft of hair and very close to the scalp, so that nits further than 1/4 or 1/2 inch are dead and may be ignored. This myth is probably largely responsible for the repeated infestations suffered among children of even the most diligent parents. *It is not true.* Researchers have seen lice lay up to three or four eggs on a shaft of hair, though one egg is more usual. And they have found viable eggs six to eight inches out from the scalp of a girl with long hair.

MYTH: nits further than 1/2 inch from the scalp are dead.

FACT: viable eggs may be found 8 inches from the scalp.

The only way to know for sure is to examine the nit closely under a magnifying glass. New viable eggs are plump and a creamy color. Empty eggshells are white. Eggs which are red or black contain a dead embryo, but if the embryo had not developed before death, the egg has a flattened collapsed appearance. Very small or deformed eggs laid by dying lice may appear after treatment. Eggshells which have been present for a very long time may be worn down to only a fragment attached to the hair.

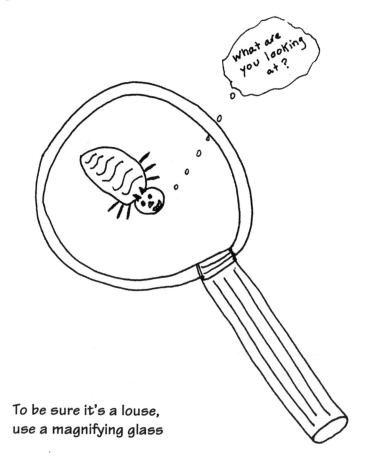

To be sure it's a louse,
use a magnifying glass

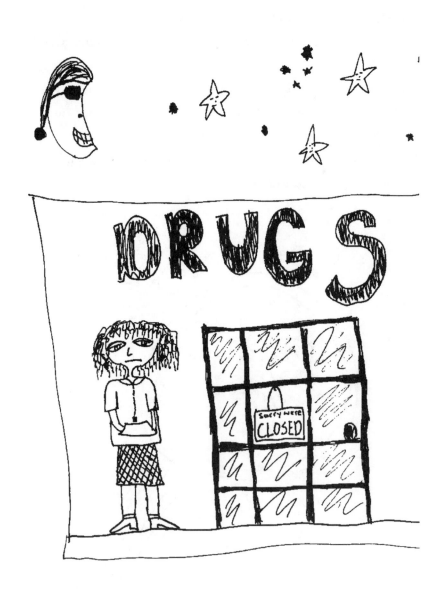

Mother seeks lice treatment — too late!

CHAPTER 3

Stalking the Wild Louse

BE PREPARED

Inevitably, you will discover lice on your child's head just after everybody's tucked into bed, it's pouring rain, and every market or drug store within miles is closed. If you have a child between 5 and 12, *be prepared. Keep in your medicine cabinet a bottle of pediculicide* — lice treatment — and a nit comb. If you already have had lice in your home, replace the used-up bottle right away. There's likely to be a next time. But check the expiration date and make a note to restock before your supply expires: treatments lose their potency over time.

SYMPTOMS

The most common symptom of a lice attack is what the doctors call pruritus and we call *itching*. However, this symptom is not always present. Up to half of children infested may not itch. Itching occurs when lice bite and suck blood from the scalp: the louse's saliva creates a reaction with the skin. If you see your child scratching his or her head often, you should check for head lice. And do it right away before lice can be spread. Do not put it off.

> Your child can have lice
> for a week before
> showing any symptoms.

After the first lice bite, a day usually goes by without any symptoms. In 24 hours, a pin point area of inflammation without itching will appear. Itching becomes intense in about a week, but in the meantime, your child may have been spreading lice throughout your home and his/her school. Eventually, the itching diminishes.

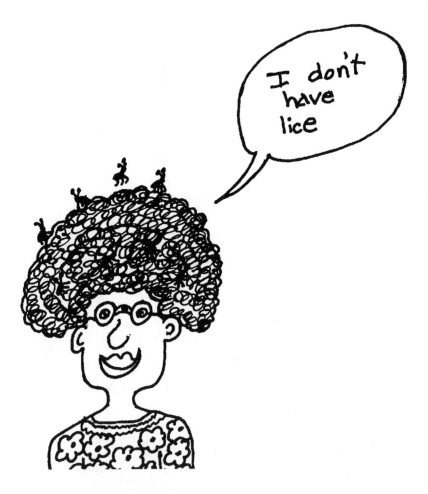

You can have lice without knowing it

In subsequent reinfestation, bites that had healed may reappear and itching become more intense when old bite sites are scratched. This means that children who have had previous lice infestations may suffer increasingly severe itching.

Close inspection of the hair and scalp with a strong light and a magnifying glass will sometimes reveal the adult lice, but you are more likely to see the nits. Sometimes other traces of lice are visible: the pinpoint red bite marks and/or small black specks of lice-poo. Fecal specks may be seen on the collar if the hair is long and the collar is light-colored. Other symptoms are swelling of the lymph glands located on the back of the neck, near the ears.

Some children may be "carriers," spreading lice while having no symptoms themselves.

LICE ALERT!

Lice are reported at school. The mother of your child's friend calls to say Johnny has lice. Maybe your daughter is scratching her head, maybe she isn't. *What do you do?*

1. Don't panic. Having head lice is not a social disgrace and not a serious problem. Lice need be no more bothersome than the common cold. Unlike the cold, lice infestations are treatable and the cure is immediate, if you follow instructions for their elimination precisely.

2. Be sensitive to your child's feelings. There is no need to scare, blame or humiliate your child. This need not be a traumatic experience. While you go through the steps below, stay calm, be supportive, and keep your sense of humor.

3. Check your child's head right away. Delay will only allow the lice to spread and create more work for you. If your child has lice and spends time lounging on your couch, pillow-fighting on your bed, or doing headstands on the carpets, you will have an intense house cleaning situation on your hands to prevent reinfestation.

4. Don't think a quick glance will do it. Stalking lice requires patience and diligence, plenty of time, and the right equipment. Don't try to do this just as your child is about to rush for the school bus or is falling asleep at bedtime! If you wait until bedtime, your child will be tired, cranky, and less cooperative. Treatment can take over an hour.

HOW TO CHECK YOUR CHILD'S HEAD FOR LICE

If you've never seen a louse, you could easily find nothing when in fact your child is infested. They are so small! Accurate diagnosis is essential for managing head lice. Here's how:

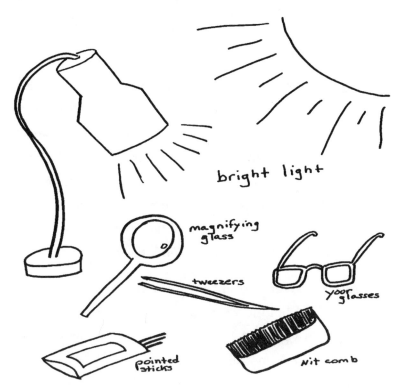

bright light

magnifying glass

tweezers

yoor glasses

pointed sticks

Nit comb

Tools needed for lice checks

Step 1. **Gather your tools:** your glasses if you wear glasses, a magnifying glass, and a pointed stick for separating the hair. A letter opener, toothpick, paint brush handle, chop sticks or any pointed object that will not scratch the scalp will do. Hair clips to separate the hair are very helpful.

Step 2. **Find a good spot** to examine your child's head: it must be comfortable, under very bright light — or better yet, natural daylight. Explain to your child that you will be examining his/her head for at least five minutes, and maybe up to fifteen minutes. Use this time to talk to your child, but keep it pleasant. (In fact, many children quite enjoy having their mothers pick through their hair. It can be very soothing if you are not hysterical.)

Step 3. **Start at the nape of the neck.** Part the hair in a straight line and scrutinize the exposed scalp. Study it for any speck. Look long enough for your eyes to focus and to spot any slight movement. Remember, lice are nearly invisible and they shy away from light. They also move quickly, but it is this nearly imperceptible movement that may catch your attention. Look specifically at the root of each hair, as lice will hide at the bottom and *behind* the hair shaft.

Step 4. **Cover the entire head in this way**, making parts 1/4 inch from the previous one and examine the scalp as in step 3. If you have reason to believe your child has lice but you haven't found any upon first examination, go over the head again.

> Looking for lice is like
> looking for a needle in a haystack,
> except that lice run and hide.

From experience I must say this: persevere. Almost every time I found lice on my kids' heads, I had searched thoroughly, decided they were lice-free, but kept going "just to be sure" or because my child was enjoying having her head scratched. And sure enough, just as I was about to quit, I would spot a nearly invisible flutter of a mere fleck — a louse scuttling between the strands of hair.

Although the instructions that come with lice treatments say look at the nape of the neck and around the ears, I have rarely found lice there: on my children they seem to prefer the top of the head and above the ears. So look everywhere. Cover all the scalp; literally, leave no hair unturned.

What about checking yourself? Your head itches. There's no adult around to go through your hair and the children are not old enough to examine your head for lice. What do you do? One simple trick that works is this: cover a desk or table with a white cloth, then, leaning over this cloth, comb your hair with a nit comb. Get the comb as close as possible to your scalp and comb all the way along the strands of hair, making sure that *anything* that falls off drops onto the cloth. If you have lice, you are likely to snag at least one of the critters in the comb and will find it wriggling on the white cloth or crawling along a fragment of broken hair. You may also discover dandruff, dirt, or gnats. To be sure it's a louse, use your magnifying glass.

If you still aren't sure whether or not you or your child has lice, you can make sure by shampooing and rinsing the shampoo into a basin and straining the rinse water through a white kitchen towel. If you or your child has lice, you will see lice on the towel. Remember, they are not necessarily dead even if they don't move — they may be faking!

NOT ALL SPECKS ARE NITS

What appear to be lice or nits may not be. Specks may be merely sand or other playground debris. And of course, there's dandruff, easily distinguished from lice by its irregular flakes and easy removal from the hair. Harder to distinguish from lice are desquamated epithelial cells (DEC plugs), small white clumps stuck to the hair shaft. These are produced by the scalp when the oil glands work overtime to compensate for dryness, often in response to excessive use of lice treatments.

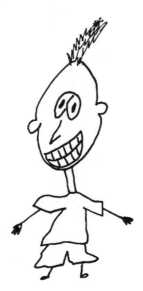

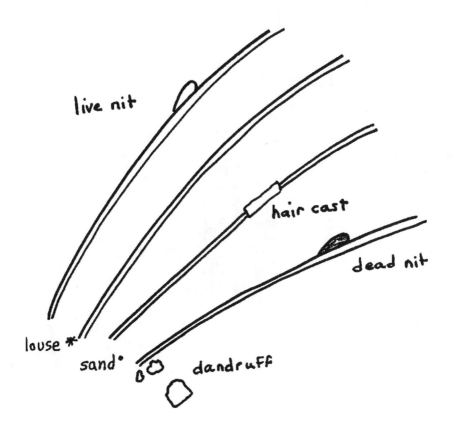

live nit

hair cast

dead nit

louse *

sand °

dandruff

Not all specks of white are lice or nits

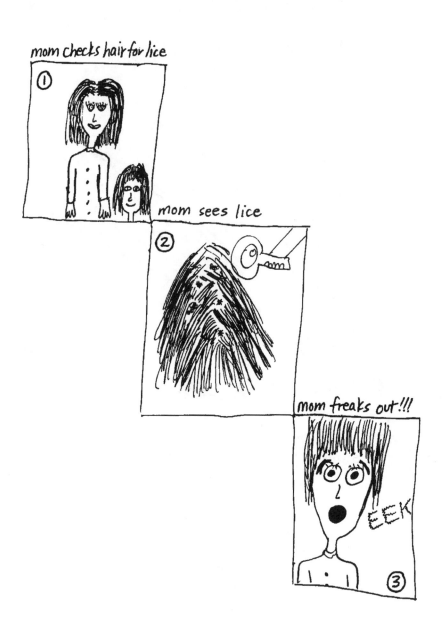

How Mom feels about lice

CHAPTER 4
EEK! Your Child Has Lice — What To Do

I FOUND ONE!

Okay, your child has lice. If you have spotted one, there's no need to look further: just one louse calls for treatment.

All family members should be examined for lice. The infested child's parents and teachers must seek another knowledgeable adult to examine their heads just as thoroughly as the child is examined. It is altogether too common that adults who have no symptoms fail to have themselves checked, yet when the child is reinfested, they point a finger at the school or another child. Many adults don't check themselves because they think they are immune to lice either because of age, hygiene, blood type, or hair treatments such as coloring or permanents. These do *not* prevent lice.

Anyone who is found to have lice must be treated. Experts recommend treating the whole family whether or not they have lice. Studies have shown that treatment is more likely to be successful when everyone is treated for lice, as opposed to only those infested being treated.

Lice treatment is a job for an adult. Do not ask your child to do this if you really want to be sure of effective treatment. In my informal study, I found that the children who applied the lice treatment themselves very quickly came down with another infestation.

HOW TO GIVE YOUR CHILD A LICE TREATMENT

Step 1. **Gather supplies:** shampoo, pediculicide, three towels, nit comb, and timer. For important information and comparison of available pediculicides, see Chapter Six. Make sure the pediculicide is not older than the expiration date because these treatments can lose their potency over time.

Step 2. **Read instructions.** Shake bottle well.

Step 3. **Remove child's clothing** and place directly in the washing machine or a sealed bag.

Step 4. **Wash child's hair with shampoo** that is water-based and high pH such as Prell, which strips the hair clean, preparing it for the pediculicide. Generally, the best shampoos for this are the cheapest. Just be sure to use a shampoo with a pH level no lower than 6 and no additives such as conditioner, protein, fruit and vegetables.

NOTE: If you will be using Nix, do *not* use hair conditioner or other substance that might block the action of the pesticide. If you want to use vinegar or products such as Clear and Step 2 to help with nit removal, apply and comb out the nits *before* you shampoo your child's head.

Step 5. **Towel dry hair.** Even if the instructions say to apply the pediculicide to wet hair, the lice treatment will be diluted if the hair is *too* wet. It should be as dry as possible from towel drying, without being completely dry. A simple test to be sure the hair is dry enough is to take a section of toilet paper and place it on your child's head. If the tissue absorbs water and sticks, the hair is too wet.

Step 6. **Cover your child's eyes** with a towel. Make sure eyes are tightly closed.

Step 7. **Treat hair in the sink.** Do *not* treat your child in a bathtub or shower. In fact, it's best *not* to treat your child *after* a hot bath or shower because the heat opens the skin and allows the pesticide to penetrate and enter the bloodstream more easily. (This is important with a product such as lindane.)

Step 8. **Apply pediculicide** undiluted to the hair until the entire scalp is covered and moistened. You may want to use rubber gloves. *Avoid inhaling.* Remember, even if prescribed by your doctor, some of these "medications" are pesticides that can have serious side effects if misused — Kwell for example. Do not assume more is better: *use only the quantity prescribed* on the bottle. If it gets in the eyes, rinse immediately with water.

NOTE: Nix has been approved for infants down to two-months old. Generally, though, do *not* use pediculicide on infants or pregnant or nursing women. Manual removal of lice and eggs is their only alternative.

Step 9. **Set your timer or alarm clock:** it is important not to exceed the time limit stated in the instructions. During this time, you can accomplish several other important tasks:

1. Inspect fingernails, both your child's and your own, for nits and lice. A louse or nit could easily become lodged beneath your fingernail. I've seen it happen.

2. Examine all household members and ask an adult to examine your head for lice or nits.

3. Call parents of children who might have been exposed to your child and ask them to check for lice or nits.

4. Do a mental inventory of the places your child might have shed lice or nits: couch, carpets, bed, etc.

5. Prepare to launder all possibly contaminated items: sheets, bedding, clothes, etc.

6. Remake the beds.

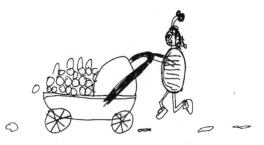

Step 10. **Rinse out the pediculicide,** when time is up. If using a treatment with residual effect (i.e., Nix), do *not* shampoo or use a conditioner or other hair products after treatment. Any such lotions will reduce the residual effectiveness of the pediculicide, which can continue to kill lice for ten days to two weeks after treatment.

Step 11. **Towel dry hair** with a new towel (not the one used before treatment). Comb damp hair thoroughly to detangle, in preparation for the fine-toothed nit comb. If you are using Nix, do not use a detangling lotion.

Step 12. **Comb hair with a nit comb** to remove dead lice and nits. Because NO lice treatment kills 100% of the nits, it is important to remove each and every nit to prevent them from hatching and reinfesting the child or family again.

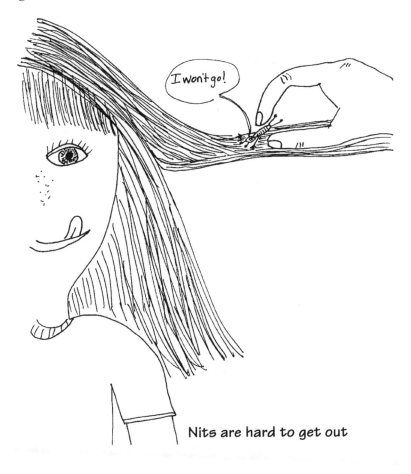

Nits are hard to get out

Nit removal is the most vital step.

Nit removal is a painstaking, time-consuming, and often very frustrating task. The nits do not come off easily: each must be snagged firmly by fingernails or lice comb, slid down the hair shaft and removed. There is nothing that dissolves the glue; there is no shortcut short of shaving the head.

Vinegar is often recommended, with dubious effect. A fairly new product called *Clear* loosens the nits to speed up the process and reduce the pain of combing tangled hair. But it does not work 100%. No product can detach *all* lice from the hair, so the parent must still go through the hair thoroughly with a good nit comb and pick out remaining nits with fingernails. If Clear is applied before or after Nix, it will inhibit the effect of the treatment; in this case, it is best to use nit removal concentrate before the Prell shampoo. If Clear is used with any of the pyrethrin lice treatments such as Rid, A-200, R&C Shampoo, or Clear Shampoo, (see Chapter 6), it should be the last step in treatment. While these treatments are less effective than Nix, they do facilitate the vital step of nit removal. It is a tradeoff, a decision only you can make based on your child's hair and temperament.

Nit removal is the step many parents fail to do completely or postpone too long. Just remember this: one remaining nit that hatches will soon lay eggs and you'll have to go through the whole procedure again!

HOW TO REMOVE NITS

First, make sure you really have a decent nit comb, i.e. one with the finest possible teeth to scrape the nits from the hair. The combs that come with lice treatments are often inadequate. Metal lice combs sold separately (such as Derbac or Medicomb) are preferable. It's good to have several on hand and use a different one for each child.

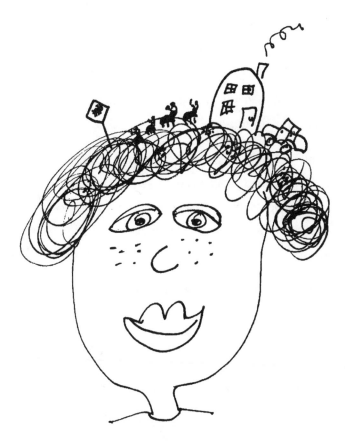

Once lice move in, they are hard to evict

USING THE NIT COMB

1. Part hair into four sections and pin with clip.

2. Pick one section and start at the top of the section.

3. Lift a one-inch wide strand of hair. With your other hand, place the teeth of the comb in the hair, as close to the scalp as possible.

4. Pull the comb firmly away from the scalp to the end of the hair. Make sure the teeth of the comb are as deep into the strand of hair as they can go. Comb all the way to the end of each strand. Resistant nits may be scraped off by backcombing the hair, especially near the scalp. Remove any remaining nits with your fingernails.

5. Using bobby pins or hair clips, pin back each strand after you have removed nits. Wipe nits from the comb often with a tissue. Dispose of each tissue in a sealed bag or flush down the toilet to avoid reinfestation. I've found it easiest to sit by the sink where I can rinse the nit comb frequently.

6. Continue until you have combed each strand in the entire section of hair.

7. Repeat these steps in the remaining sections of hair.

8. If the hair dries, dampen slightly with water.

9. After combing the entire head, rinse thoroughly.

10. After hair is dry, recheck the entire head for stray nits and remove them.

11. Have your child put on clean clothes that cannot possibly have been exposed to lice.

AFTER THE TREATMENT

It's worth repeating: no pediculicide is 100% effective, even those that claim to kill all lice and eggs. It may be impossible to remove absolutely all the nits, so it's wise to repeat treatment in one to two weeks, depending on the package instructions, to kill any remaining nits which may have hatched. But most brands of lice treatment suggest not doing more than two consecutive applications within 24 hours.

Head lice can become resistant to pediculicides. If treatment is unsuccessful, check whether the label directions were followed carefully. If so, use another pediculicide with a different active ingredient.

LICE IN EYELASHES OR EYEBROWS

Rarely, lice are found in the eyelashes and eyebrows. Never apply a pediculicide around the eye area. The lice and/or nits will have to be picked off one by one and disposed of, or obtain an ophthalmic ointment from your pediatrician. This vaseline-type substance will need to stay on your child's eyelashes about 24 hours to suffocate lice.

TREATMENT FOR ITCHY SCALP

Virtually nothing topical has been found to relieve the itching caused by lice bites, though some say itching may be relieved by a warm baking soda bath. Since the itch caused by lice bites are an allergic reaction, antihistamine pills may help.

Thursday Plantation Tea Tree Oil (melaleuca alternifolia) and Tea Tree Oil shampoo and conditioner have been found by some parents to be effective in soothing all kinds of itching, including lice bites. However, lice experts say it is ineffective, highly allergenic and not recommended. I don't know. If you use it, rinse it off quickly if the scalp begins to burn.

I have discovered that *ice packs* work best with all itches, but it took my children a while to accept the cold on their heads. You can make an ice compress child-friendly by covering it in a thin piece of material with a child's print or your child's favorite cartoon character.

In any case, scratching must be discouraged as it will make the itch worse and possibly spread bacteria. In four to five days the itch should subside.

COOPERATION

Inform your child's teacher and the parents of any friends with whom he/she has had recent contact. Advise them to check their own children to prevent further spread

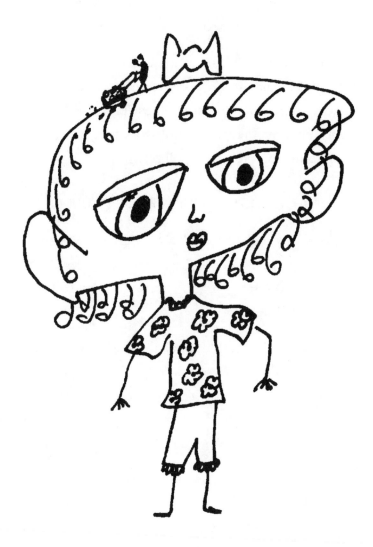

Just one remaining nit may hatch and start
a new infestation

of lice. The school may want to put out an alert to other parents to check their children and to ask those infested to remain home until treated and lice/nit free.

This kind of communication and cooperation is essential because pediculosis is a social disease. Lice are spread by contact. To get control over an infestation, it is important that parents, children and the school work together. (See Chapter 8 for information on school policies.)

"OH NO, NOT AGAIN!" THE DIFFICULT CASE

You can't believe it. You've tried everything. Nothing works. Your child *still* has lice. You can't take it any more. You swear, you are going to shave your child's head or run away from home.

Now, calm down. It's not all that bad. Not as bad as those sleepless weeks when your newborn little darling woke you every few hours for feeding. Somehow, you got through it. Try to think of lice as just one more diaper, one more scraped knee, one more temper tantrum. They come with the package.

Now that you are calm, think back. And be honest with yourself. Did you really remove all the nits? Did you reapply the pediculicide after 7 to 10 days as instructed on the package? When you applied the treatment, had you thoroughly towel-dried your child's hair or was your child's hair wet, hence diluting the medication? Are you sure you covered the entire head, or did your child squirm so much that you may have missed a spot? Did you wash your child's hats, clothes and linen? Have you instructed your child in ways to avoid reinfestation from others at school? Have you done everything listed in this chapter and Chapter 5?

If you can answer yes to all these questions, there is a treatment of last resort. When all else fails, treat your child with Nix but this time, after towel-drying the hair and making sure the Nix completely covers the scalp and hair, *leave it on for an hour.* Rinse thoroughly and meticulously comb out the nits. This is sure to work and it is perfectly safe. Other products with higher concentrations of permethrin are safely left on the skin for longer periods of time — for example, Elemit, a 5% permethrin cream used in the treatment of scabies. Leaving Nix on longer than the prescribed ten minutes is not recommended in normal cases of lice because Nix properly applied *works* in ten minutes and generally it is unsound practice to use more of any medication than necessary.

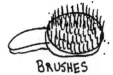

HEAD BANDS

HATS

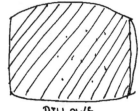

BRUSHES

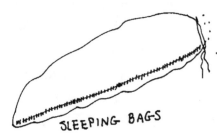

SLEEPING BAGS

PILLOWS

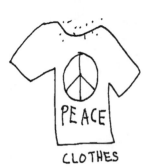

PEACE

CLOTHES

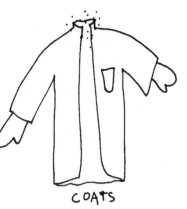

COATS

How lice travel

CHAPTER 5
Your Lousy Home

DON'T BE BUGGED

After you have treated your child and members of the household, you must delouse the house, unless you discovered the lice during the trip back from camp and your child has not stepped foot in your home. In that case, drop off the camp gear at the cleaners and immediately upon arrival home throw your child's clothing into the washer and treat your child for lice.

More likely your child has been wandering around your home for days, shedding hair that may have carried lice or nits everywhere. These wandering lice and hatching nits may reinfest your child and infest the whole family.

Delousing your home does *not* mean a frantic, back-breaking disinfecting of everything in the house. Studies have shown that with proper treatment of the infected child and his/her contacts, cleaning the home is virtually unnecessary and does not warrant the expense and effort many parents put into washing, dry cleaning, and storage. The point is to take the extra precaution of eliminating lice from areas and items where the infested person might have shed lice or nit-carrying hairs. For those that can manage it, a fine alternative is simply to leave the house for a week to ten days. During that time any nits will hatch and the lice will die. Of course, this only works for those who can afford it and only if you don't take any lice or nits with you.

PUT ON THE HEAT

The best way to kill lice is with heat. You don't need to boil lice, though rest assured, boiling would do the job. You can delouse items by immersion in hot water at 50 degrees centigrade for 30 minutes or 60 degrees centigrade for 10 minutes. Lice can also be killed by hot air. It would take one hour exposure to still air at a temperature of 70 degrees centigrade to kill a louse, though the time can be reduced by air circulation.

Lice are also affected by cold, and in laboratory conditions, lice and nits will die at a temperature −20 degrees centigrade for five hours or −15 degrees centigrade for ten hours. But killing nits on your clothing or bedding will require longer exposure to lower temperatures because the fabric insulates and protects them from the cold.

COMBS

Family combs and brushes must be treated. Don't forget combs in other parts of the house, such as the guest bathroom, your handbag and the car. Treatment options include:

1. Scrub your combs and brushes and remove all hairs;

2. Heat in water over 60 degrees centigrade (150 degrees Fahrenheit) for ten minutes;

3. Soak in pediculicide for a day or two;

4. Microwave for a minimum of 2 minutes.

Beware that boiling water may damage combs and brushes. The microwave is likely to melt plastic and burn fabric before it kills lice. I've seen a louse crawl merrily across a baseball cap as the hat curled to a crisp in the microwave oven. And remember, do not put metal in the microwave, for example, the tiny metal clip on pony tail bands.

Keep in mind that using pediculicide to delouse combs and brushes is not a 100% guarantee the nits will be killed, just as it is not a guarantee on the head. (See Chapter 6.)

LINENS AND CLOTHING

Anything which may have been exposed to your child within the last week should be considered a possible lice motel, a stopover between hosts. These items must be treated.

Wash bed linens and washable clothing in hot water at least 150 degrees Fahrenheit and dry in a hot dryer for at least 20 minutes. Lice and nits may also be killed by putting dry fabrics in a clothes dryer on hot cycle (155 degrees Fahrenheit) for 20 minutes.

Most washers don't give temperatures, so how can you be sure the water is hot enough? One way is to check your water heater, if it has a gauge. Or dip a thermometer into a cup of hot water.

While the laundry is washing, take a moment to delouse your laundry basket. Don't use it again until it has been deloused.

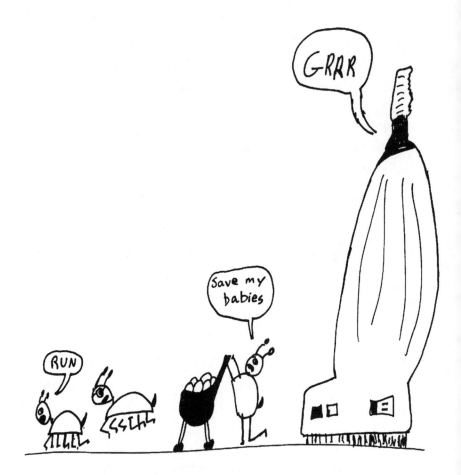

Don't forget to vacuum

VACUUM

Carefully vacuum mattresses, sofas, chairs, pillows, carpets and other furniture that might have been exposed to the hair and lice of the infested person. Empty or dispose of the vacuum bag.

You may also want to use the hose attachment to vacuum coats in the coat closet, particularly around the neck, and clothing hanging in the closets of all infested family members.

Likewise, it makes sense to vacuum toys, particularly stuffed animals, that your child has spent time with just before the infestation.

HOT IRON

Ironing with a hot iron is another effective way to rid fabrics of lice, especially material not washable or easily dry cleaned. Use the hot iron around seams of sofas, pillows, stuffed animals, and the like.

SPRAYS

Insecticide use in the home is controversial. The National Pediculosis Association is firmly against sprays and in 1988 the Centers for Disease Control reported that lice remedies in their vaporous state (i.e., sprays) are more harmful than liquid formulations because they are more readily absorbed through the lungs.

Dr. John Becher of the National Center for Infectious Disease, Department of Health and Human Services, has stated: "There is no evidence that the use of environmental insecticides in an institution or home achieves faster control of head lice than no use of insecticides at all." He added, "Although insecticides, when properly used, are generally safe and effective, the tendency towards abuse of these products and the possible environmental hazards caused by such abuse are, in my opinion, greater than the health hazards posed by lice."

If you feel you must use an insecticide spray, be sure to use only lice spray and do not spray humans or pets. Spray only sofas, carpets and other household items than cannot be laundered or dry-cleaned. (For example, do not spray your child's pillow.) Read and follow the directions on the can. Provide good ventilation and avoid inhaling the spray. Allow items to dry completely before using.

BAGGING

Personal items and clothing that cannot be washed at high temperatures or dry-cleaned should be isolated in a plastic bag for ten days. During this time the nits will hatch out and die. When ready, open the bag outdoors and shake out each item vigorously.

If the article is your child's favorite blanket or stuffed animal, you may not want to remove it during this traumatic episode. Instead, vacuum or iron it and inspect it carefully for lice, nits or your child's hair which may carry lice or nits.

DON'T FORGET THE CAR

The car, especially if used in a car pool, is a frequently overlooked haven for lice. Vacuum the car thoroughly.

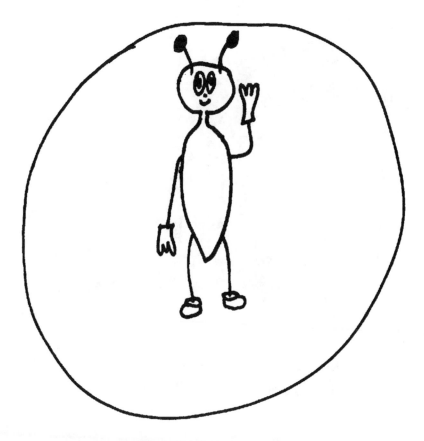

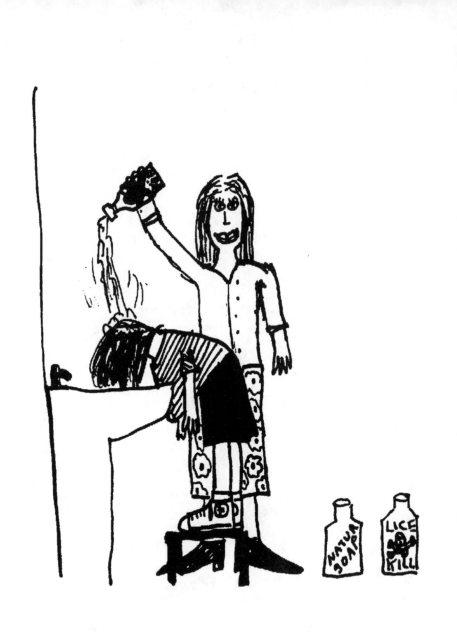

Misuse of lice treatments may be
hazardous to your child's health

CHAPTER 6

Treatment Options: Think Twice About What You Put On Your Child's Head

Historically, head lice have been controlled by DDT, malathion, carbaryl, kerosene with olive oil, and other concoctions. Not only have several of these treatments been found to be extremely toxic, but lice seem to have developed resistance to some of them. Resistance ultimately threatens all types of control by conventional insecticides, so we are faced with the ever-challenging task of finding alternative measures which are lethal to lice but not harmful to people.

Several chemically unrelated ectoparasiticides are available to treat pediculosis. In order of preference they are:

PERMETHRIN

Permethrin (Nix) is a synthetically developed compound that has been found to be superior to all other lice treatments. Not only does it have a higher lice and nit fatality upon treatment than any other product, it also has residual activity lasting for 10 days to two weeks, killing lice hatching after the treatment. Permethrin is non-toxic, has low absorption into the skin, and few side effects. Safety in nursing and pregnant women and infants under the age of two months has not been established.

Nix is a 1% permethrin cream rinse — the only permethrin product on the market. It is applied to the hair after shampooing and left for ten minutes before rinsing out. It leaves the hair glossy and manageable. The hair should not be shampooed for 24 hours after treatment.

Tests show that permethrin can kill all lice and 99% of the nits in one application. However these tests were conducted by trained personnel who applied the treatment precisely as required and under optimum conditions. In the general population where real parents apply the treatment in varying ways, the "cure rate" would probably be closer to 70% or 80% — still more effective than any of its competitors. The implications are clear: follow instructions precisely and reapply again in 7 to 10 days.

PYRETHRINS

Popular over-the-counter lice treatment products (except Nix) nearly all contain pyrethrins as the active ingredient. These are natural products derived from the chysanthemum. Pyrethrins include Rid, R&C Shampoo, Triple X liquid, A-200 Pyrinate, Lice-Enz, Pronto, Tisit, Lice-trol. They are safe and effective, but they are highly photo-unstable and lose their potency within 12–24 hours after exposure to light.

Because pyrethrins lack residual activity, they are no longer effective after the treatment so any nits that hatch soon after treatment will live. For this reason, it is especially important to comb out all nits and to reapply the treatment after seven to ten days.

Pyrethrins may aggravate asthma and allergies in persons sensitive to ragweed pollen or chrysanthemums. For highly sensitive individuals, pyrethrins can provoke life-threatening allergic reactions. The FDA warns that the product:

(1) should not be used by persons sensitive to ragweed;

(2) should not be inhaled;

(3) should not be swallowed;

(4) should not be used near the eyes;

(5) should not be allowed to come in contact with mucous membranes, i.e., the eyes, nose or mouth.

LINDANE

Lindane is the active ingredient in products such as Kwell and its generic equivalents. Lindane is prescribed by doctors not because it is more effective than other treatments (it isn't) but because it is too dangerous to be sold over the counter. In fact, lindane has been shown to be possibly the *least* effective of commercial remedies in terms of time needed to kill adult lice and percentage of eggs surviving after treatment (30%). Many people believe lice have become resistant to lindane, but this medication was never effective to start with. Because lindane does a poor job of killing lice, it must be applied again a week later to kill newly hatched nymphs — doubling the exposure to a toxic substance.

Lindane is expensive and has more side effects than other treatments. Its misuse can cause rash, contact dermatitis, conjunctivitis, aplastic anemia, leukemia, central nervous system damage, hematological (blood) disorders, cornea damage, seizures, and acute poisoning. Inhalation can cause headaches, nausea, irritation of eyes, nose and throat. Finally, lindane may be carcinogenic, and misused, lindane may be lethal. The Environmental Protection Agency has suggested that lindane be banned.

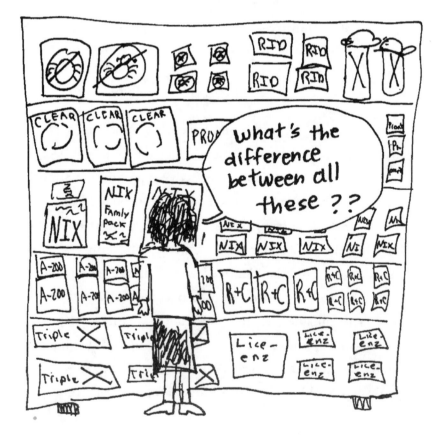

The manufacturers of lindane claim the product is "safe when used as directed," but directions are incomplete, instructions from the doctor and pharmacists may be inconsistent, and the presence of lice is so discombobulating that many parents apply the shampoo incorrectly. For example, parents may apply lindane in the bath or shower (since it is called a "shampoo"); they may leave it on for 10 minutes (like other pediculicides); and they may use the whole bottle instead of the directed one teaspoon (some doctors prescribe 4 teaspoons) because one teaspoon cannot begin to cover the scalp or saturate the hair.

One mother who took her convulsing child to the emergency room after a Kwell treatment reported to the doctor that the child had not been exposed to any type of toxin: it never occurred to her that the prescribed medication, a "shampoo," was a pesticide.

Take note: As this book was going to press, I received notice that the manufacturers of Kwell have stopped producing it. Kwell will be available only as long as supplies last. However, generic lindane and other brands containing lindane may be around for some time. For any prescribed lice treatment, be sure to ask your pediatrician and/or pharmacist if lindane is the active ingredient. If it is, ask for something else.

MALATHION

Malathion, once the treatment of choice, is no longer recommended. It is highly effective against both lice and the eggs but it is also extremely unpleasant and highly flammable. When used, it is applied for 8–12 hours and patients must avoid hair dryers, flames, and burning objects such as cigarettes during treatments.

NATURAL TREATMENTS

Rumor suggests that some natural/herbal shampoos prevent lice infestations and can be used to treat lice infestions. However, none have been properly tested or shown to be effective. None have been FDA approved for treatment of lice.

Thursday Plantation claims its Tea Tree Oil shampoo and conditioner helps control head lice. Although the company is unable to produce any concrete evidence, it has testimonials from customers who claim Tea Tree Oil was the only thing that worked to finally eliminate lice that had not responded to other treatments. I tried it and it didn't work.

If you decide to try tea tree oil, here's what you do: add 20 drops (1/2 to 1 tsp) of pure tea tree oil to a handful of tea tree oil shampoo. Apply this mixture to the head. After ten minutes, rinse and comb the hair thoroughly with a nit comb to remove nits. Repeat this treatment the next day and two times a week until clear of nits. Of course, this rigorous nit-picking is likely to be responsible for the effectiveness of the treatment.

I have found a concoction that actually works, even on chronically infested kids on whom all other treatments have failed. I hesitate to recommend it because, as far as I know, it has not been scientifically tested, and I cannot vouch for its safety. I include the recipe with this warning: *do not assume that ingredients are not toxic simply because they are "natural."* The essential oils below are highly concentrated and may be toxic if not diluted and even lethal if taken internally. They must be diluted per instructions. Pennyroyal oil is not recommended for pregnant women — it is used to cause abortions.

Alternative Recipe
$1/2$ teaspoon pennyroyal oil
$1/2$ teaspoon eucalyptus oil
$1/2$ teaspoon rosemary oil
8 teaspoons extra virgin olive oil

Stir together the ingredients. Shampoo your child's hair, towel dry, and apply the oil mixture as you would any treatment (see pages 34 and 35). Saturate the scalp and hair: girls with long hair may need to increase the recipe.

Tie the hair under a shower cap secured with a bandana or head band so that the cap will not slip. Caution: oil may cause color to run. Use a hair covering that will not bleed. Keep the mixture on overnight. In the morning, shampoo and remove all nits.

Idea: The three essential oils above are all insect repellents. Perhaps a drop or two of this recipe on your child's hair before going to school may help prevent reinfestation.

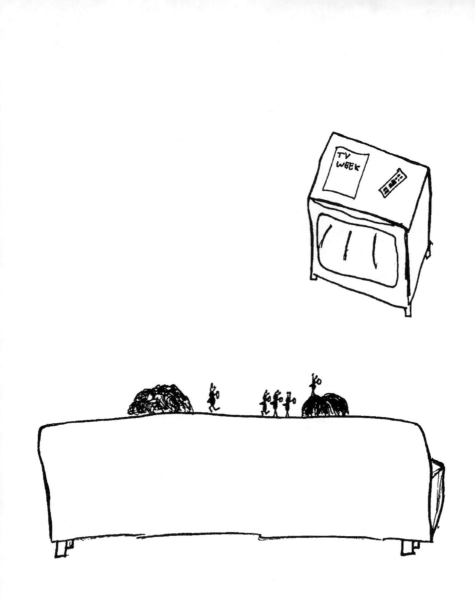

Sharing more than a moment together

CHAPTER 7

Prevention Is Worth a Pound of Pediculicide

SAY "NO" TO BUGS

Head lice can cause great physical discomfort and emotional distress for the child, and infestations can be a major annoyance for parents in time and effort. As if the hassle weren't enough, there is the cost. A family of four can spend in one infestation the following:

Treatment

Nix 4 bottles @ $11.95	$47.80
Prell 1 bottle	3.99
lice combs 4 @ $4.29	17.16
pediculicide spray 3 @ $4.29	12.87

Dry cleaning

sleeping bags 2 @ $16.95	$33.90
comforters 4 @ $27.90	111.60
blankets 4 @ $22.95	91.80
TOTAL	**$319.12**

In addition to the $319 out-of-pocket expenses is the cost of washing at home 4 sets of linens, 12 towels, 1 bathmat, 4 jackets and countless items of clothing. Lice treatment is not only an ordeal for the family, it's expensive. Repeated infestations and the failure to gain control over the problem become a significant financial burden.

BASIC PREVENTION

Controlling head lice requires an understanding of how they are spread. Remember, they generally are passed from child to child or from child to parent or teacher. Head lice cannot fly or jump, they can only crawl. There are some things you can do to minimize the risk of your child contracting head lice. First and foremost is teaching your child to avoid the kinds of contact that allow lice to spread. Discuss each of these points with your children:

1. Don't borrow combs, brushes, barrettes, hair ribbons, or other personal items.

2. Don't share or borrow hats, helmets, scarves, pillows or sleeping bags.

3. Hang hats and coats separate from others, not one on top of another. Hats can be tucked into pockets or coat sleeves. Jackets could also be kept in a knapsack.

4. If sharing earphones, headphones, or sports equipment head gear, check them carefully and clean before using them.

5. Avoid putting heads together with other children during lice alerts.

6. Never pick up or wear any hat or clothing found on the street or elsewhere.

7. Wash any clothing retrieved from lost-and-found before wearing.

TRICKS OF THE TRADE

Parents with years of experience with lice have contrived a number of tricks to deal with them. Here are just a few ideas:

• Insist that any child with long hair wear braids or pony tails, or otherwise keep their hair tied back and "unavailable" to lice.

• Check your children's heads immediately upon return from school, before they contaminate the house.

• Check your children's heads frequently. You may also find cause to diplomatically check his/her friend's head too, particularly before a sleep-over.

• Keep children in their own beds or sleeping bags. Do not lend or borrow bedding of any kind.

• Remove all extraneous pillows and stuffed animals from your children's beds and playroom during "lice season." This way, you'll have less to deal with when lice invade your home.

- Provide each member of the family with personal towels and do not share.

- Hang your children's hats and coats on a separate hook in their own rooms, not in the downstairs "guest" closet or coat rack.

- If you are unable to treat your child immediately, cover his/her head with a hair covering such as shower cap, ski hat, surgical cap and the like. Make sure all hair is tucked in and the cap is secure. Or, without punitive overtones, restrict your child to one room or one area of the house (with entertainment or homework) until you can treat. Don't keep him/her there too long!

- Similarly, if it's late by the time you get around to treating your own head, and you just can't bear to change all the bedding, wear a hair covering yourself. When you get up, you can go through the housecleaning steps you couldn't face the night before. Wash or throw the hair covering away.

- If lice seem to be a chronic problem, keep accessible a change of linen, pillows, blankets, or sleeping bag to simplify the change of bedding when you discover lice on your child. Also have back-up combs and brushes.

- Never trust your child or his/her teacher or camp counselor with the report that your child does not have lice. *Check for lice yourself.* Many professionals don't know how to conduct a lice check and their examination of large numbers of children may be perfunctory. (The last time my child reported "They checked me at camp," I found about 20 lice on her head and spent the day shampooing and house cleaning.)

THE PLACES WE DON'T THINK ABOUT

On airplanes: those little white paper napkins folded over the headrest are there for a reason, originally to prevent spread of head lice. But they may not be changed with each turn-over of passengers, so ask the flight attendant for a new one or place your own handkerchief, bandanna or scarf over the headrest. You may want to do this in buses and taxis during "lice season" too.

In carpools: collaborate with participating drivers to assure the upholstery in the car is lice free. In a serious outbreak, mothers might agree to check the kids' heads before getting into the car.

Movie theaters are an overlooked source for lice contagion. Every two to three hours a new person slumps down in each seat, squirms about a good deal, and sheds hair (and possibly lice and nits) on the upholstery. To play it safe, go to the first show of the day. Chances are any lice deposited the day before will have died or wandered off the back of the seat. Brush off your seat where your head or hair might touch, and cover the back of the chair with a scarf, sweatshirt or jacket that you do not plan to wear upon leaving the theater.

In waiting rooms, avoid resting your head on the chairs or couches — especially the pediatrician's office, dentist chair, child psychiatrist, library and the like where plenty of children pass through and camp out for a while on the furniture. This would include the school lobby and school principal's office!

Trying on clothing: try to make sure your child tries on items that have *not* been tried on by someone else previously. This may be hard to control and there is no evidence to suggest transmission via clothing stores, but it's a remote possibility. Be particularly careful when trying on hats.

THE PQRST'S OF LICE CONTROL

Be prepared: Have lice treatments on hand.

Be quick: Respond to lice alerts immediately.

Be responsible: Tell anyone with whom
your child has had contact.

Be safe: Apply treatment according to instructions.

Be thorough: Remove all nits and treat your home for lice and nits to prevent reinfestation.

Be prepared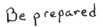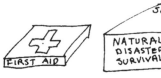

Be quick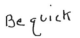

Be responsible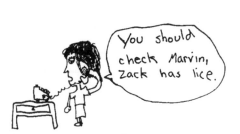

Be safe

Be thorough

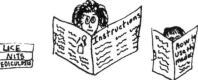

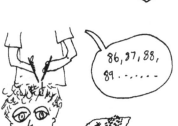

The PQRST's of lice control

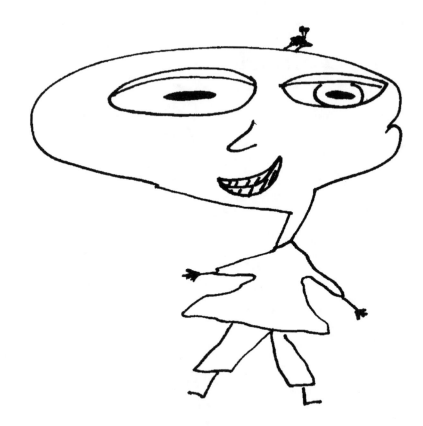

CHAPTER 8

Questions Frequently Asked About Lice

1. If my child washed her hair more often, would that reduce her chances of getting lice?

No. Personal cleanliness does not prevent a person from getting head lice.

2. Are lice carriers of AIDS?

No one knows for sure. Some suspect they could be simply because lice do puncture the skin and their saliva enters the blood stream, but it is unlikely.

3. I've heard that a larger, faster moving breed of lice is invading the U.S. Is it true?

There is no evidence of a new breed of lice. One California health official made the observation of a larger louse, but when the louse was sent to a lab, it was found to be a body louse, not a head louse. Adult head lice can be up to 3mm long.

4. Can head lice jump or fly?

No. They crawl and they prefer to crawl along a shaft of hair rather than striking out onto another surface. If a child should shed that strand of hair and it lands on another child's head (e.g. in a shared hat, comb, or carpet where the kids are playing, the louse can quickly move to the second child's hair and make a new home for itself.

5. Why do some kids seem never to get them while others suffer infestation after infestation?

Nobody knows for sure. However, it appears that blood type may play a role. Preliminary studies at the University of Miami indicate that lice may have difficulty moving from a person of one bloodtype to someone with another bloodtype.

6. If my child gets head lice, should I cut her hair?

Not necessarily. Long hair will not predispose her to getting lice, it will only make it harder for you to deal with the lice treatment and to remove the nits.

7. Every parent and every doctor seems to have differing and sometimes conflicting information about lice. Are there any "experts" in lice treatment that can advise us?

You are right: many doctors, including pediatricians, don't know much about lice or lice treatment. Many pharmacists would be a better source of information. There are experts, but only a few in the U.S. Unfortunately their research is severely under-funded.

8. Why do some parents allow their children to go to school or someone else's home when they know the child has lice?

Some parents are embarrassed and don't know what to do about lice. You could share your concern with those parents or ask the school to meet with them. Or, you could diplomatically give them this book. Other parents believe the lice are a lesser problem than the lice treatment and refuse to put toxins on their children's heads. These parents must be urged to use other methods, i.e., methodical, manual removal of every lice and nit from their child's head. It is not fair to subject a community to lice. Lice control is possible only when everyone cooperates. You may want to urge your children's school to institute a "no-nit" policy which would keep out children whose parents inadequately respond to the problem.

9. I just finished thoroughly delousing the house. And now the lice are back — do I have to clean house again?

Sorry to say, the answer is, yes. If you have caught this second lice infestation before your child has wandered around contaminating your freshly cleaned home, you need only wash those items/areas that might have been exposed to this new batch of lice. On the other hand, if it's possible that you missed something in the house cleaning, you might want to go through the whole procedure again.

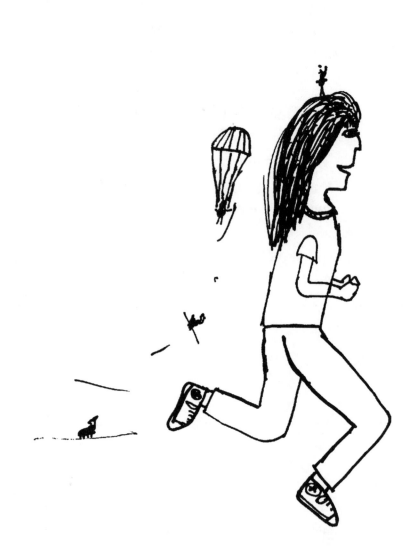

We shed hair wherever we go

10. What about pets? Could my dog or cats be "carriers?"

Lice do not live and breed on any animal except the human. Still, your pets could be temporary hosts just like a hat or pillow upon which your child's hair has fallen. We shed hair all day long, everywhere we go, so if your child is around the pets, chances are the animals could receive a stray hair or louse. This does not mean the pets should be treated; a good check and brushing should do.

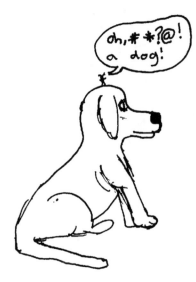
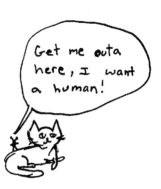

Pets do not harbor lice

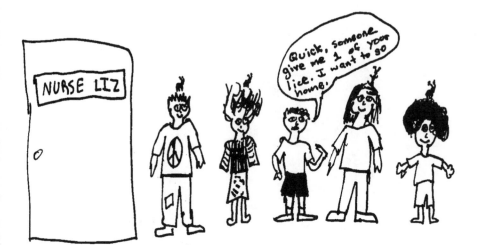

Children found to have lice are sent home

CHAPTER 9

Special Information for Schools

Prevention and control of head lice outbreaks is dependent upon early detection, effective control measures, and education. Every school should establish a lice policy and communicate that policy to teachers, staff and parents.

Education is important because many people are misinformed about lice. A study commissioned by Burroughs Wellcome and performed by the Princeton Opinion Research Inc. found in a phone survey of 1022 Americans over the age of 18 that 50% would be embarrassed by head lice in the family, 25% thought lice are a problem for the poor or dirty, 35% believed pets transmit lice and 46% believed a hair cut is necessary to control lice. My own survey revealed that many parents are simply not aware of the treatment steps that are necessary to eliminate lice. Intelligence, education, income and career success do not equip parents for dealing with lice.

At the beginning of each school year, and periodically thereafter when lice appear, the school should instruct children in the facts of head lice transmission and encourage students to take appropriate precautions. No, that is not enough. *"Encourage"* is inadequate if lice are to be controlled. Just like prohibitions against hitting or littering, rules relating to lice must become part of the school culture. Preventive measures must be mandatory and enforced, including:

1. No sharing combs, brushes, and other hair grooming items.

2. No exchanging clothing that has been worn, and in particular, no swapping hats.

3. Wiping clean headgear, head phones, and the like before use.

4. No sitting close together with heads touching.

5. Hanging coats so they don't touch others.

6. No sharing sleeping bags or mats at naptime; no sleeping close together with heads touching.

7. No sharing costumes and no use of wigs.

8. Staying home if known to have lice.

SCREENING

A screening program should be instituted at the beginning of each school year in the vulnerable age groups (ages 5–12). The school should announce the dates of these checks in advance to parents. After the initial screening, conduct periodic checks. If a large school population has to be screened it may wise to invest in a Wood's Light which makes lice detection easier.

During the initial and subsequent screenings, all children present should be checked, and any children not present should be checked when they return to school. Siblings of children found to have lice should also be checked.

It is standard policy in many schools that *any child found to have live lice is sent home.* An alternative would be to have the parent come to the school and treat the child right there if this can be done without embarrassing the child. After treatment, nit-combing and a change of clothes, the

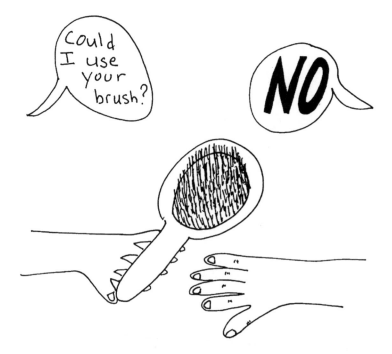

Don't borrow combs, brushes, hats or sleeping bags

child should be returned to the classroom and reintegrated into school activities without disruption or undue attention. If the child is cared for by a nanny during work hours, that person should be trained in lice treatment and asked to treat the child.

If the rule is that children with lice must be sent home, they should be sent home with a minimum of fuss. The parents of the child should be provided with clear instructions for lice treatment (or this book) and instructed that the child will not be permitted to return to school until lice treatment has been performed and the child is lice and nit free. The child and his/her siblings should be examined at the school upon his/her return and allowed to stay only if found to be completely free of lice and nits.

Any child found to have *nits but no live lice* should be examined more carefully to determine if the nits are "fresh" or old and dead. (See Chapter 2 for a description of the difference.) If the nits are dead, the child can be returned to the class room. If the nits are alive, some schools allow the child to stay in class and to return home at the end of the day with instructions to the parents to treat the child. This is a mistake: where there are nits there are certain to be live lice. Children with live nits should be sent home until treated and found to be nit-free.

INSPECT THE FACILITY

Sometimes something in the school allows lice infestation to become chronic. A walk through the buildings and classrooms may reveal trouble spots. Observe specifically the places and ways in which the students heads and hair come into contact, directly or indirectly. Where do they rest their heads? Also look for all the places their clothes are intermingled or in close contact. Sometimes the activities need to be considered, i.e., dress-up play time especially in the lower pre-school and kindergarten levels.

GUIDELINES

Schools that are serious about eliminating lice follow these guidelines:

1. Assign children individual lockers or coathooks spaced so that the clothes of other children do not touch. Lice infestations are higher in classrooms where children share storage space for personal belongings.

2. If individual hooks are close together, have each child put his/her coat on the back of their assigned seats, with scarves and hats placed into the sleeves of their garments.

3. Do not allow coats and hats to be piled up, for example, outside the gymnasium, on the front steps of the school, etc.

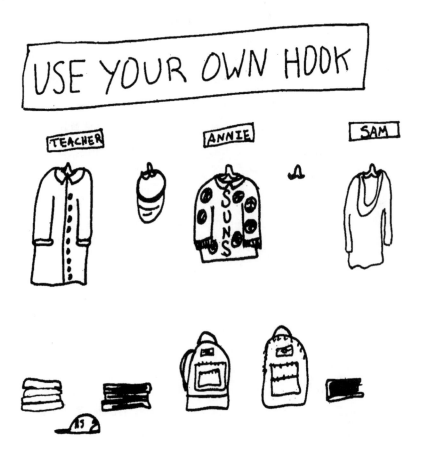

USE YOUR OWN HOOK

TEACHER   ANNIE   SAM

Hang coats apart from each other

4. Assign sports clothing, helmets and equipment for the game season and store these items in individual lockers. They should be washed frequently — and certainly washed if any child is found to have lice.

5. Reconsider the use of head phones and other head gear during a lice alert. If they must be used, they should be wiped clean after each student and spraying should be considered.

6. Dress-up corners should be discontinued during lice outbreaks. Consider alternatives to children sharing these clothes. Use disposable articles if possible. Certainly avoid wigs and other headgear.

7. Remove furniture or toys that might be harboring lice and nits. In one school, a large stuffed bear that all the kids climbed on and cuddled in turned out to be a Grand Central Station for lice.

8. During an outbreak, eliminate classroom activities involving close physical contact or the wearing of costumes or hats.

9. Vacuum carpeted classrooms daily.

10. Permanently assign resting mats or pillows and keep them separated while in use as well as during storage. They should not be stacked together, but should be in separate bags for storage and laundered frequently. Mats should be wiped clean regularly.

WHEN LICE ARE A CHRONIC PROBLEM

Lancet, the prestigious medical research magazine, reported findings some time ago that indicated the only way to really control a lice outbreak is to treat everybody. This suggests that when lice become a serious problem in any school, the entire school must cooperate.

One day may be selected to be a day *every child* in the school will be treated at home, *whether or not they have lice or nits*. That same day the school will implement an overall lice deinfestation program of spraying, vacuuming, removing stuffed animals and costumes, laundering sports equipment, and the like.

When lice are a chronic problem, the parents can become exceedingly distraught. Sometimes those who complain the most about "others" spreading lice are the ones who aren't exactly following the precise lice treatment requirements themselves. Fingers are pointed in all directions. It's important that all parents be adequately informed and urged to take steps to delouse their child and the whole family.

To make sure parents are adequately knowledgeable about the control of head lice, the school should consider hosting an evening seminar, complete with demonstration, and urge all parents in the vulnerable age groups to attend.

JURISDICTIONAL DISPUTES

Where there are no-nit policies, it's not uncommon for school officials and parents to disagree about whether or not the child has lice and must go home. The argument comes from a knowledge gap. Many people who *should* know what lice look like don't, but that doesn't necessarily stop them from having a strong opinion. Dr. Juranek of the Centers for Disease Control tells the story of a priest who suspended a large number of kids from school because they had lice. Asked how he knew, he said, "I could see them jumping from head to head." This is clearly a man who doesn't know lice don't jump and can barely be seen, even close up, much less across a room!

The issue is, who decides? If the parents see no lice and the pediatrician sees no lice but the teacher knows that he/she sees lice: who determines the fate of the child? It can be difficult when the parties to the dispute all consider themselves experts.

No one solution could apply to all school districts. In some areas it might be the school principal, in others the district nurse. More important is, first, adequate education about lice to assure that all the obvious personnel really can recognize a louse, and second, the proper equipment to make a diagnosis: specifically, a good magnifying glass.

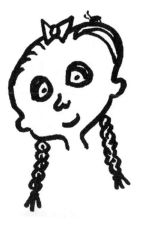

"Hey, ask me!"

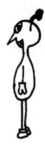

"Trust me, I can help..."

"I know all about lice!"

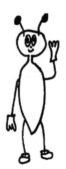

CHAPTER 10

Resources

ORGANIZATIONS

National Pediculosis Association
P.O. Box 149, Newton, Massachusetts 02161
tel: (617) 449-NITS

The NPA newsletter, *Progress*, provides up to date news on lice treatment, research, side effects of pesticides, lawsuits, etc.

VIDEOTAPES

Barney Barks about Head Lice, produced by Smith Kline Beecham. A puppet dog explains away kids fears and answers questions about lice. Distributed by Modern Talking Picture Service, Inc.

LITERATURE

There is very little written about lice. Two books interesting from a historical point of view might be in your library:

Zinsser, Hans, *Rats, Lice and History*, 1935
Buxton, Patrick A., *The Louse*, 1939

You should have better luck in medical libraries, although these books are technical and often out of date regarding treatment of lice:

Alexander, John O'Donel, *Arthropods and Human Skin*, Springer-Verlag, NY, 1984.

Lehane, *Biology of Blood-Sucking Insects*, Harper Collins Academic, London, 1991

Orkin, Milton, Howard Maibach, Lawrence Parish, and Robert Schwartzman, *Scabies and Pediculosis*, J.B. Lippincott, Philadelphia, 1977

Rook, Arthur and Dawber, Rodney, *Diseases of the Hair and Scalp*, Blackwell Scientific Publications, Boston, 1982

Round Table discussion at Harvard on *Pediculosis Management, a Guide for the '90s.*

Lice Treatment Checklist

_____ check all members of family for lice or nits

_____ wash hair with shampoo like Prell
(use no conditioner)

_____ apply lice treatment, following instructions precisely

_____ remove all nits

_____ delouse combs, brushes, head bands, hats, etc.

_____ launder sheets, pillow cases, clothing

_____ hot dry or dry clean blankets, bedspreads, etc.

_____ vacuum carpets and furniture

_____ wipe clean car upholstery

_____ inform school and parents of others in contact
with your child

_____ retreat in 7 days

_____ inspect hair every three days during lice season
or lice alerts

ORDER FORM

Please send THE LICE-BUSTER BOOK to:

Name _____

Position _____

Organization _____

Address_____

Purchase Order Number _____

Price: $9.95 per book x _____ = $_____
                                 QUANTITY

Less 10% Discount for orders of 100 or more $_____
For orders over 500, call 415-381-3551

Subtotal $_____

Sales tax: Add 7.75% for books
shipped to California addresses $_____

Shipping and handling:
Air Mail: $4.50 per book $_____
Book rate: $3.50 for one book;
       75 cents for each additional $_____
     (Surface shipping may take three to four weeks.)

TOTAL $_____

Payment:
Please make check payable to *Authentic Pictures* and mail to
Authentic Pictures, 89 Walnut Avenue, Mill Valley, CA 94941

Fax Orders:
Fax Order Form and Purchase Order to (415) 381-2469

For further information, call Authentic Pictures, (415) 381-3551